Enoxaparin (Clexane) & Pregnancy

How Necessary and Safe is It?

Asharani Sah

Enoxaparin (Clexane)
&
Pregnancy

How Necessary and Safe is It?

Author: Asharani Sah
Published by: Self-Published
Publisher Address: Bihar, India

First Edition

ISBN: 978-93-342-4679-7

Dedication

To **Lord Shri Ramakrishna,**

whose wisdom inspires the pursuit of
knowledge and the service of humanity.

Preface

Blood clots can be life-threatening, and **Enoxaparin (Clexane)** has become a vital medication in the **prevention and treatment of Deep Vein Thrombosis (DVT), Pulmonary Embolism (PE), and clot-related complications in pregnancy and surgery**. Despite its widespread use, many patients and caregivers find themselves overwhelmed with questions about how Enoxaparin works, how to use it safely, and what precautions are necessary.

This book, **"Enoxaparin (Clexane) and Pregnancy: How Necessary and Safe Is It?"**, is designed to be a **comprehensive yet easy-to-understand** guide for patients, caregivers, and anyone seeking reliable information about this essential anticoagulant. Unlike complex medical textbooks, this book explains **the uses, dosage, side effects, precautions, and real-world applications** of Enoxaparin in **simple, accessible language**—whether you are taking it yourself or caring for a loved one.

What You'll Learn in This Book:

✓ **Step-by-step instructions** on how to safely inject Enoxaparin at home

✓ **Answers to common concerns** about dosage, side effects, and lifestyle adjustments

✓ **A quick-reference guide** for emergency situations, side effects, and dosage charts

✓ **Special considerations** for pregnancy, surgery, and long-term use

This book is not a substitute for professional medical advice, but a **trusted companion** to help you feel more confident and informed while managing your health with Enoxaparin (Clexane). Whether you're a patient, caregiver, or simply looking for **clear, research-backed information**, this guide will serve as a **valuable resource** on your journey toward better health.

📌 **Stay informed. Stay safe. Take charge of your health.**

Table of Content

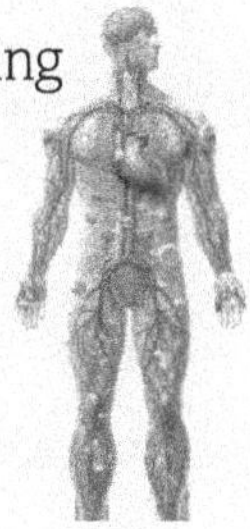

--------Disclaimer---------

This book is intended for educational and informational purposes only and should not be considered a substitute for professional medical advice, diagnosis, or treatment. Healthcare providers should always exercise clinical judgment and refer to the latest medical guidelines before prescribing Enoxaparin (Clexane) or any other medication.

Every effort has been made to ensure the accuracy and reliability of the information presented. However, medical science is constantly evolving, and new research may provide updated insights. This book does not claim to be comprehensive or definitive, nor should it be relied upon as the sole source for clinical decision-making.

The author, Asharani Sah, does not endorse or promote any specific tests, treatments, physicians, pharmaceutical products, or medical procedures mentioned in this book. Readers are strongly encouraged to consult with qualified healthcare professionals for any medical concerns or treatment decisions.

Chapter 1:
Understanding Enoxaparin (Clexane)

What Is Enoxaparin?

Enoxaparin, commonly known by its brand name **Clexane**, is a medication used to prevent and treat blood clots. It belongs to a class of drugs called **low molecular weight heparins (LMWHs)**, which are derived from heparin, a natural substance in the body that helps prevent clotting. Enoxaparin works by interfering with the blood's ability to form clots, reducing the risk of serious conditions like deep vein thrombosis (DVT), pulmonary embolism (PE), and strokes.

Brand Names and Forms (Injections, Prefilled Syringes)

Enoxaparin is available under different brand names worldwide, with Clexane being one of the most commonly used. Other brands may include **Lonopin, Lovenox,** and **Inhixa**, depending on the country.

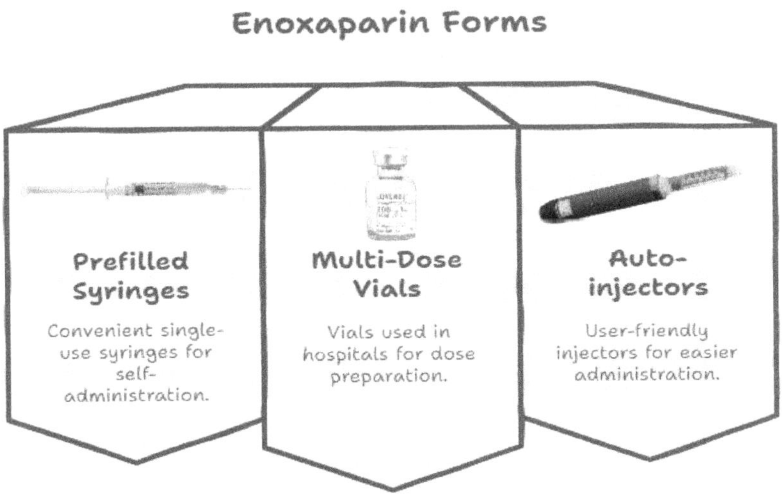

1. **Prefilled Syringes**: These are the most common and convenient form. Each syringe contains a pre-measured dose of enoxaparin, making it easy for patients to self-administer at home. The syringes are designed for single use and are available in different strengths (e.g., 20 mg, 40 mg, 60 mg, 80 mg, or 100 mg).
2. **Multi-Dose Vials**: These are less common and are typically used in hospital settings. They require a healthcare professional to draw the correct dose into a syringe before administration.
3. **Auto-injectors or pens** (available in some brands for easier use)

The medication is usually injected **subcutaneously** (under the skin), often in the abdomen, thigh, or upper arm. The prefilled syringes are designed to minimize discomfort, with thin needles and clear instructions for use.

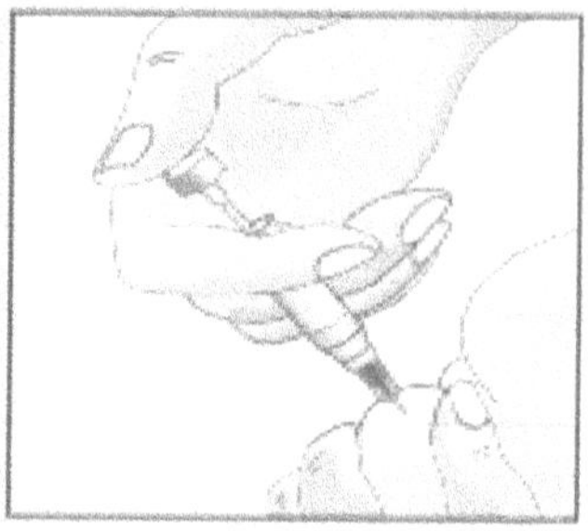

What Conditions Does It Treat?

Enoxaparin is prescribed to prevent and treat a variety of conditions related to blood clots. These include:

1. Anticoagulation in Pregnancy

Enoxaparin (Clexane) is sometimes prescribed during pregnancy to manage clotting risks and support maternal and foetal health. While pregnancy is a natural state, certain conditions increase the risk of blood clots, which can threaten both the mother and baby. Enoxaparin, a low molecular weight heparin (LMWH), is often preferred in pregnancy because it does not cross the placenta, making it safer for the developing foetus compared to other anticoagulants like warfarin.

2. **Deep Vein Thrombosis (DVT)**:

DVT occurs when a blood clot forms in a deep vein, usually in the legs. If left untreated, the clot can break loose and travel to the lungs, causing a life-threatening condition called pulmonary embolism (PE). Enoxaparin helps prevent the formation of these clots or stops existing clots from growing larger.

3. **Pulmonary Embolism (PE)**:

PE is a serious condition where a blood clot blocks one of the arteries in the lungs. Enoxaparin is used to treat PE and prevent further clots from forming.

4. **Preventing Clots After Surgery**:

Patients undergoing certain surgeries, such as hip or knee replacement, are at high risk of developing blood clots. Enoxaparin is often prescribed to reduce this risk during recovery.

5. **Unstable Angina and Heart Attacks**:

Enoxaparin is sometimes used in patients with unstable angina (chest pain caused by reduced blood flow to the heart) or heart attacks to prevent further clotting in the coronary arteries.

6. **Preventing Clots in Hospitalized Patients**:
Patients who are bedridden or have limited mobility due to illness are at risk of developing blood clots. Enoxaparin may be used to prevent clots in these situations.

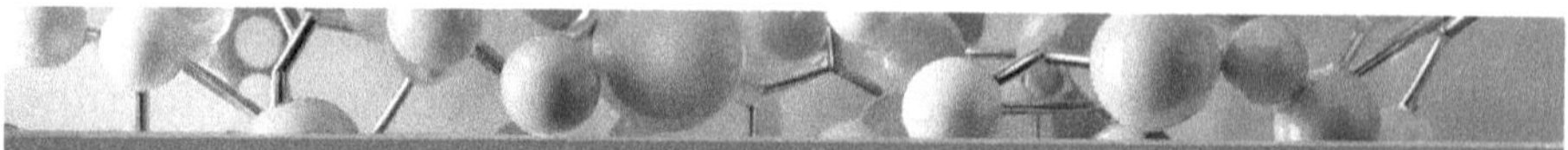

HOW DOES ENOXAPARIN WORK?

The Science Simplified: Blood Clot Prevention

Enoxaparin (Clexane) is a powerful medication that helps prevent and treat blood clots, but how does it actually work? To understand this, let's break down the science into simple terms.

The Basics of Blood Clotting

Blood clotting, or coagulation, is a natural process that helps your body stop bleeding when you're injured. However, when clots form inside blood vessels without an injury, they can block blood flow and cause serious health problems. These unwanted clots can lead to conditions like deep vein thrombosis (DVT), pulmonary embolism (PE), or even strokes.

The clotting process involves a series of steps and relies on proteins in your blood called **clotting factors**. One key player in this process is **thrombin**, an enzyme that helps convert a protein called **fibrinogen** into **fibrin**. Fibrin forms a mesh-like structure that traps blood cells, creating a clot.

How Enoxaparin Intervenes

Enoxaparin belongs to a class of medications called **low molecular weight heparins (LMWHs)**. It works by targeting a specific clotting factor called **Factor Xa** (pronounced "Factor Ten-A"). Here's how it helps:

1. **Inhibits Factor Xa:**
    - Factor Xa is a critical enzyme in the clotting cascade. It helps produce thrombin, which, as mentioned, is essential for clot formation.
    - Enoxaparin binds to a natural substance in your blood called **antithrombin III**. This binding enhances antithrombin III's ability to block Factor Xa, effectively slowing down the clotting process.
2. **Prevents Clot Formation:**
    - By inhibiting Factor Xa, enoxaparin reduces the production of thrombin. This, in turn, limits the formation of fibrin, the mesh-like structure that forms clots.
    - As a result, enoxaparin helps prevent new clots from forming and stops existing clots from growing larger.

Why Enoxaparin is Unique

- **Predictable Effect:** Unlike older blood thinners like unfractionated heparin, enoxaparin has a more predictable effect on the body. This means doctors can prescribe it without needing to monitor blood levels as frequently.
- **Longer-Lasting:** Enoxaparin stays active in the body for a longer time, allowing for once- or twice-daily dosing.
- **Targeted Action:** It specifically targets Factor Xa, reducing the risk of excessive bleeding compared to medications that affect multiple clotting factors.

Chapter 2:

When Is Enoxaparin Prescribed?

Enoxaparin (Clexane) is widely used for **preventing and treating blood clots** in various medical conditions. Doctors prescribe it when there is a **high risk of clot formation**, which could lead to serious complications like **deep vein thrombosis (DVT), pulmonary embolism (PE), heart attacks, or pregnancy-related clotting disorders**.

1. **Pregnancy**
   - **Why Prescribed:** Pregnancy increases the risk of blood clots due to hormonal changes, reduced mobility, and pressure on blood vessels. Women with clotting disorders (e.g., thrombophilia), a history of recurrent miscarriages, or preeclampsia may be prescribed enoxaparin to ensure a safe pregnancy.

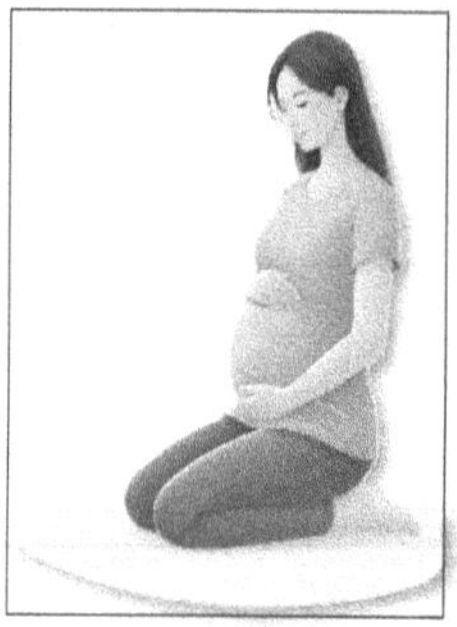

   - **How It Helps:**
     - **Preventing Pregnancy Loss:** In women with clotting disorders like antiphospholipid syndrome or Factor V Leiden, blood clots can form in the placenta, disrupting blood flow to the foetus and leading to miscarriage. Enoxaparin prevents these clots, improving the chances of a successful pregnancy.

- **General Clot Prevention:** Enoxaparin also prevents clots in maternal veins, reducing the risk of complications like deep vein thrombosis (DVT) or pulmonary embolism (PE) during pregnancy.

- **Key Point:** Enoxaparin is safe during pregnancy because it does not cross the placenta, making it a preferred choice over other blood thinners like warfarin.

2. **Deep Vein Thrombosis (DVT)**

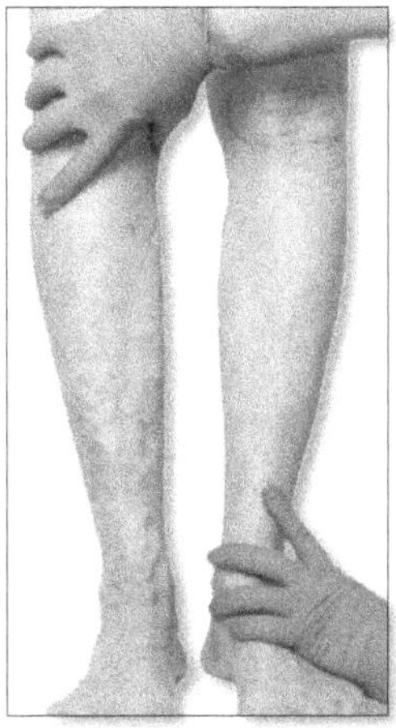

Enoxaparin is widely used to treat and prevent DVT, a condition where blood clots form in the deep veins, usually in the legs. DVT can lead to serious complications if the clot dislodges and travels to the lungs, causing a pulmonary embolism. Enoxaparin helps by reducing the blood's ability to clot, thereby preventing the formation and growth of clots.

3. **Pulmonary Embolism (PE)**

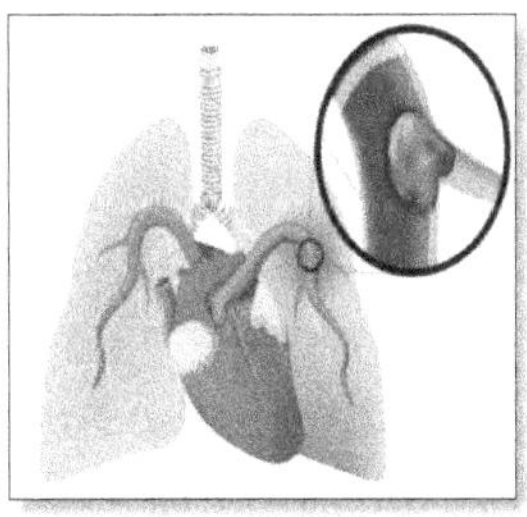

Pulmonary embolism is a life-threatening condition where a blood clot blocks one or more arteries in the lungs. Enoxaparin is used to treat and prevent PE by inhibiting clot formation and promoting the breakdown of existing clots. It is often administered in the acute phase of PE treatment and may be continued for a period to prevent recurrence.

4. Heart Conditions (Angina, Heart Attacks)

Enoxaparin is often prescribed for **heart-related conditions** where blood clots can block arteries supplying the heart. These include:

- **Unstable Angina:** A condition where the heart doesn't get enough blood due to **partial artery blockage**.
- **Heart Attack (Myocardial Infarction):** When a clot completely blocks a heart artery, cutting off blood supply.

- **Stent or Angioplasty Procedures:** After heart surgery, **Enoxaparin prevents clot formation in stents or bypass grafts**.

How It Helps:

☑ Prevents clots that can trigger a heart attack
☑ Improves blood flow to the heart
☑ Reduces the risk of stroke or secondary heart attacks

Heart patients often take **Enoxaparin in combination with aspirin or other blood thinners** for added protection.

5. Post-Surgery Prevention

After major surgery, **patients are at high risk of blood clot formation** due to prolonged immobility and changes in blood circulation. Enoxaparin is commonly used after:

✔ **Orthopedic Surgeries:** Hip or knee replacements carry a high risk of DVT and PE.

✔ **Abdominal or Cancer Surgeries:** Patients recovering from major operations may need **short-term Enoxaparin therapy** to prevent clots.

✔ **Hospitalization with Limited Mobility:** Patients on **bed rest** due to illness or injury may receive Enoxaparin injections as a preventive measure.

How It Helps:

✅ Reduces the risk of post-surgical blood clots
✅ Prevents dangerous clots in the lungs (PE)
✅ Allows safer recovery for high-risk patients

In surgical patients, **Enoxaparin is usually started 12–24 hours after surgery** and continued for **several days to weeks**, depending on the patient's condition.

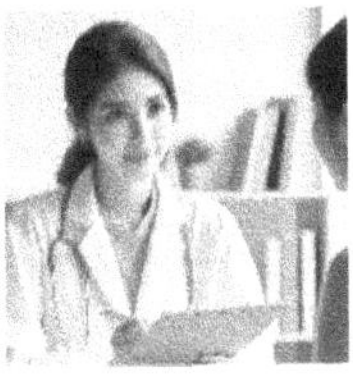

Why Doctors Choose Enoxaparin Over Other Blood Thinners

When it comes to **preventing and treating blood clots**, several anticoagulants (blood thinners) are available, including **warfarin, heparin, and newer direct oral anticoagulants (DOACs)** like rivaroxaban and apixaban. However, **Enoxaparin (Clexane)** is often the **preferred choice** in many medical situations. Here's why:

1. More Predictable and Reliable Effect

Unlike **unfractionated heparin (UFH)** or **warfarin**, which require **frequent blood tests to monitor clotting levels (INR tests), Enoxaparin has a more predictable anticoagulant effect**. This means:

☑ **No need for frequent blood monitoring** (except in special cases)

☑ **Lower risk of dose fluctuations**

☑ **Consistent and reliable effect on clot prevention**

This makes Enoxaparin **more convenient for both doctors and patients** compared to traditional blood thinners like warfarin.

2. Longer-Lasting Action, Fewer Doses

Enoxaparin has a **longer half-life** than unfractionated heparin, meaning it stays active in the body **for a longer time**. As a result:

✔ **Once or twice-daily injections** are usually sufficient

✔ **No need for continuous IV infusions** (as with UFH)

✔ **Less hospital time for patients** who need anticoagulation therapy

This is especially helpful for **pregnant women, post-surgery patients, and those recovering at home** who need a simple and effective blood thinner.

3. Safer for Pregnancy and Breastfeeding

Many blood thinners, such as warfarin and some DOACs, **are not safe for pregnant women** because they can cross the placenta and **harm the baby**. In contrast:

◆ **Enoxaparin does not cross the placenta**, making it **safe for both the mother and baby**.

◆ It is the **first-choice anticoagulant** for women with a history of **pregnancy loss, clotting disorders, or preeclampsia**.

◆ It is **safe for breastfeeding mothers**, unlike warfarin, which can have unpredictable effects.

This makes Enoxaparin **the gold standard for pregnancy-related clot prevention**.

4. Lower Risk of Major Bleeding

While all blood thinners **increase the risk of bleeding**, studies show that **Enoxaparin has a lower risk of major bleeding complications** compared to:

⚠ **Warfarin**, which requires strict INR monitoring to avoid excessive bleeding
⚠ **Unfractionated heparin**, which can cause **heparin-induced thrombocytopenia (HIT)**, a severe drop in platelets
⚠ **DOACs**, which may not have effective reversal agents in emergencies

Enoxaparin's safety profile makes it **a preferred choice for high-risk patients**, including those **undergoing surgery, with kidney disease, or with recent trauma**.

5. Trusted for Hospital and Home Use

Enoxaparin is highly versatile—it can be **used in hospitals or self-administered at home**. Unlike unfractionated heparin, which requires **IV administration and hospital monitoring**, Enoxaparin can be:

✔ **Given as an easy subcutaneous (under-the-skin) injection**
✔ **Self-injected by patients at home** after proper training

✔ **Used safely for long-term anticoagulation**

This **reduces hospital stays and costs**, making it a **patient-friendly option**.

6. Effective Across Multiple Conditions

Enoxaparin is widely used in **many medical situations**, including:

- **Pregnancy-related clot prevention**
- **Deep Vein Thrombosis (DVT) and Pulmonary Embolism (PE)**
- **Post-surgical clot prevention (orthopedic, abdominal, and cancer surgeries)**
- **Heart conditions like unstable angina and heart attacks**

Its **broad range of applications** makes it the **go-to anticoagulant** for many doctors.

Chapter 3:

Dosage Guidelines

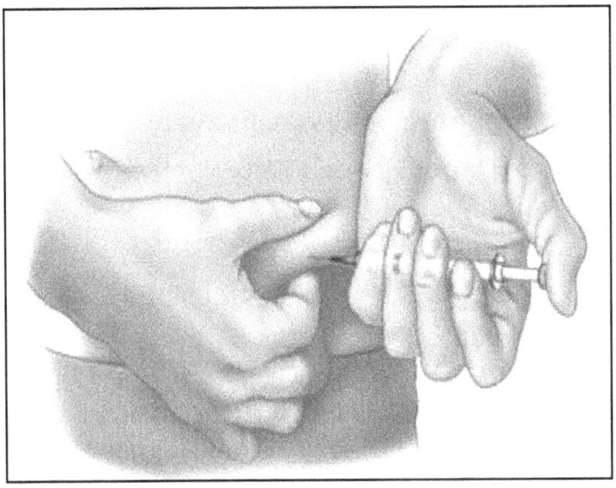

Enoxaparin is typically given as a **subcutaneous (under-the-skin) injection** in the abdomen or thigh. The dose depends on whether it is being used for **treatment (to dissolve an existing clot) or prevention (to stop clots from forming).**

Typical Doses for Different Conditions

1. Blood Clot Prevention (DVT/PE Prophylaxis)

This applies to patients at high risk of clot formation, such as **those recovering from surgery, bedridden patients, or pregnant women with clotting disorders**.

Standard Preventive Dose:

✔ **40 mg once daily** OR

✔ **30 mg twice daily** (for high-risk patients, such as those after hip or knee replacement surgery)

Duration:

✅ **7–10 days after surgery** (may extend to 4 weeks after major orthopedic surgeries)

✅ **Throughout pregnancy for high-risk women**

2. Deep Vein Thrombosis (DVT) or Pulmonary Embolism (PE) Treatment

Patients with an active **DVT or PE** require **higher doses** to break down clots and prevent further complications.

💉 **Standard Treatment Dose:**

✔ **1 mg per kg body weight every 12 hours** OR

✔ **1.5 mg per kg once daily** (for less severe cases)

📅 **Duration:**

✅ **5–10 days**, followed by oral blood thinners (e.g., warfarin or DOACs) for long-term therapy.

3. Enoxaparin Use in Pregnancy

Pregnant women with **a history of miscarriage, thrombophilia, or previous clots** may need Enoxaparin **throughout pregnancy** to prevent clot formation in the placenta.

💉 **Standard Dose for Pregnancy:**

✔ **40 mg once daily** (for prevention)

✔ **1 mg/kg every 12 hours** (for treatment of existing clots)

📅 **Duration:**

✅ **Until 36 weeks of pregnancy**, then switched to shorter-acting heparin before delivery.

4. Heart Conditions (Angina, Heart Attack Prevention, Post-Stent Placement)

Enoxaparin is used in heart patients to **prevent clot formation in arteries**, reducing the risk of heart attacks.

Standard Cardiac Dose:

✔ **1 mg/kg every 12 hours**

✔ Used in combination with **aspirin** for better protection.

Duration:

Typically **2–8 days**, depending on the patient's condition.

Enoxaparin Dosage

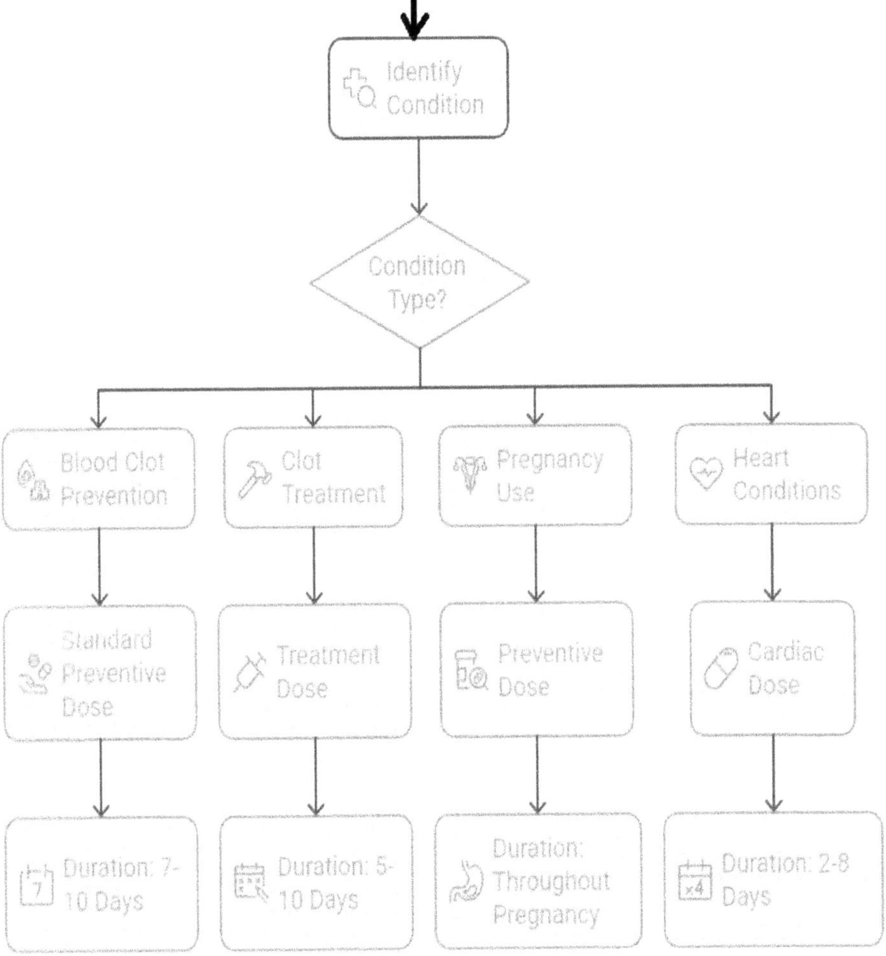

Adjustments for Kidney/Liver Issues

Patients with **kidney or liver disease** require special dose adjustments to avoid excessive drug accumulation, which **increases the risk of bleeding**.

1. Dosage Adjustments for Kidney Disease (Renal Impairment)

The kidneys help eliminate Enoxaparin from the body. **Patients with kidney disease** (low creatinine clearance) process the drug more slowly, so lower doses are required.

💉 **For mild to moderate kidney disease (eGFR 30–50 mL/min):**
✔ **Monitor closely, but no major dose adjustment is usually needed.**

💉 **For severe kidney disease (eGFR <30 mL/min):**
✔ **Prophylaxis dose: 30 mg once daily** instead of 40 mg.
✔ **Treatment dose: 1 mg/kg once daily** instead of twice daily.

🚨 **Patients on dialysis should NOT take Enoxaparin unless advised by a specialist.**

2. Dosage Adjustments for Liver Disease

Liver disease can affect **blood clotting balance**, making dosing tricky. **Patients with severe liver problems** should have:

✔ **Regular blood clotting tests (INR, APTT, platelet count)**
✔ **Lower doses if liver function is severely compromised**
✔ **Close monitoring for bleeding or excessive bruising**

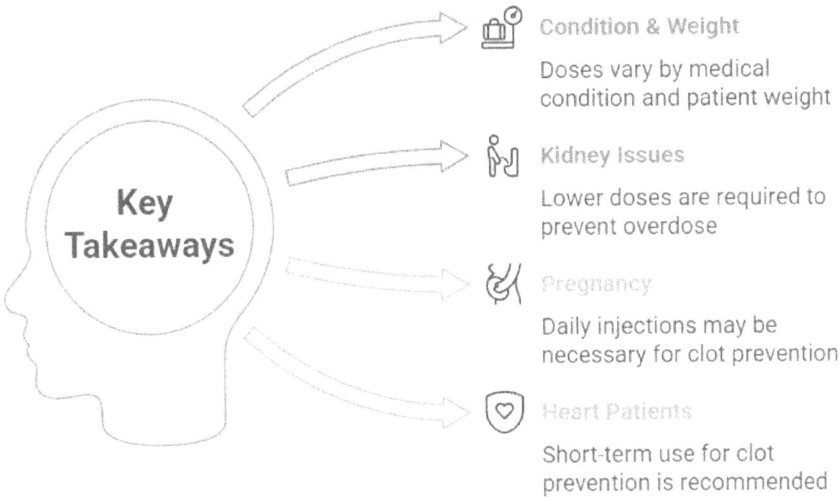

Step-by-Step Injection Guide

Enoxaparin (Clexane) is usually self-administered at home through a subcutaneous (under-the-skin) injection. Proper technique is essential to ensure effective absorption and minimize pain or bruising.

This section provides a clear, step-by-step guide to help patients confidently inject Enoxaparin at home.

How to Inject Enoxaparin at Home (With Visual Tips)

Before You Start:

✔ **Wash your hands thoroughly** with soap and water.

✔ **Find a clean, well-lit space** to perform the injection.

✔ **Gather your supplies:**

- Enoxaparin prefilled syringe
- Alcohol swab
- Sharps disposal container

✔ **Choose an appropriate injection site** (abdomen, thigh, or arm).

◆ **Step-by-Step Injection Instructions**

Step 1: Prepare the Syringe

Remove the Enoxaparin prefilled syringe from its packaging.
Hold the syringe by the body (not the plunger).
Do **NOT** push out the tiny air bubble inside—it helps ensure the full dose is administered.

Step 2: Choose and Clean the Injection Site

Where to Inject?
Best Sites: Lower abdomen, outer thigh, or upper arm.
Avoid: Areas with bruises, scars, or irritation.

Pro Tip: The **abdomen is the most recommended site** because it provides consistent absorption.

How to Clean the Skin:
✔ Use an **alcohol swab** to clean the area.
✔ Let the skin dry completely before injecting (prevents stinging).

Step 3: Pinch the Skin and Insert the Needle

Using your non-dominant hand, pinch a small fold of skin (to ensure the medication is injected into fat, not muscle).

Hold the syringe like a pen or dart at a **90-degree angle** (straight in) for the abdomen or **45-degree angle** for the thigh or arm.

✔ Insert the needle quickly but smoothly—this helps reduce discomfort.

Step 4: Inject the Medication

Slowly press the plunger all the way down to inject the medication.

Hold the syringe in place for **5–10 seconds** to ensure full delivery.

Do NOT rub the injection site—this can cause bruising.

Step 5: Remove the Needle and Dispose of the Syringe

- **Gently pull the needle out at the same angle it was inserted.**
- **Activate the safety shield** (if using a safety syringe).
- **Dispose of the used syringe** in a **sharps container** (never in regular trash).

Where to Inject: Abdomen, Thigh, or Arm?

1. Abdomen (Most Recommended)

Preferred site due to **best absorption** and fewer side effects.

Inject at least **2 inches (5 cm) away from the belly button**.

Avoid **bruised or scarred areas**.

📍 **2. Outer Thigh**

✅ Good alternative for people uncomfortable with **abdominal injections**.

✅ Pinch a thick fold of skin before injecting.

📍 **3. Upper Arm**

✅ Least common site but an option for those who cannot use the abdomen or thigh.

✅ Requires **assistance** if self-injecting.

Quick Tips for a Painless Injection

✔ **Use a new site each time** to avoid soreness and skin hardening.

✔ **Inject slowly** to reduce discomfort.

✔ **Never rub the site**—gently press with a cotton ball if needed.

✔ **Use an ice pack before injection** if you experience pain.

Storage and Handling

Proper storage and handling of Enoxaparin (Clexane) ensure that the medication remains **effective and safe to use**. Exposure to extreme temperatures or improper handling can reduce its potency or cause complications. This section covers **how to store syringes at home and travel safely with Enoxaparin.**

Keeping Syringes Safe

General Storage Guidelines:

✔ Store Enoxaparin **at room temperature (below 25°C or 77°F)**.

✔ Keep syringes in **their original packaging** to protect them from light.

✔ Do **not freeze** or refrigerate, as extreme cold can damage the medication.

✔ Keep out of reach of **children and pets**.

What If Enoxaparin Was Exposed to Heat or Cold?

Do NOT use Enoxaparin if:

✖ It was frozen or left in direct sunlight for an extended time.

✖ The liquid appears **cloudy, discolored, or contains particles**.

✖ The syringe or vial is **damaged or leaking**.

◆ If you're unsure about the medication's safety, consult a **pharmacist or doctor** before use.

Disposing of Used Syringes Safely

Used Enoxaparin syringes must be disposed of properly to **prevent injury and contamination**.

Safe Disposal Steps:

✔ **Use a sharps container** to discard syringes—never throw them in regular trash.

✔ If a sharps container is unavailable, use a **thick plastic bottle**

(e.g., detergent bottle) with a secure lid.

✔ Check local **pharmacy or hospital disposal programs** for proper syringe disposal.

Traveling with Enoxaparin

Whether you're **traveling for work, vacation, or visiting family**, carrying Enoxaparin safely is important to **ensure you don't miss any doses**.

Packing Enoxaparin for Travel

🧳 **Carry it in your hand luggage** (to prevent exposure to extreme temperatures in cargo).

◆ Keep syringes in **original labeled packaging** for easy identification.

◆ Pack a **small sharps container** for safe disposal of used syringes.

◆ Bring **extra doses** in case of unexpected delays.

Flying with Enoxaparin: TSA and Airline Guidelines

✔ **Medical syringes are allowed on flights**, but inform security officers during screening.

✔ Carry a **doctor's prescription or medical certificate** to avoid issues at customs.

✔ Store medication in a **clear plastic bag** for easy security checks.

✔ If traveling to a **different time zone**, adjust your injection schedule accordingly.

Chapter 4:

Possible Side Effects

Enoxaparin (Clexane) is generally **safe and well-tolerated**, but like all medications, it can cause **side effects**. Most side effects are **mild and manageable**, but some may require **immediate medical attention**. This chapter covers **common and serious side effects**, along with tips on how to manage them at home.

Common Side Effects

Most people using Enoxaparin experience **mild side effects** that do not require medical intervention. These typically improve as your body adjusts to the medication.

1. Bruising and Pain at the Injection Site

◇ Small bruises around the injection site are **normal** due to Enoxaparin's blood-thinning effects.
◇ Mild **redness, swelling, or tenderness** may also occur.

💡 **How to Reduce Bruising and Pain:**
✔ Alternate **injection sites** to avoid skin irritation.
✔ Use **gentle pressure** after injecting instead of rubbing.
✔ **Inject slowly** to reduce discomfort.
✔ Apply a **cold compress** to the area after injection.

2. Mild Bleeding

Because Enoxaparin **prevents blood clots**, minor bleeding (e.g., **longer bleeding from cuts or nosebleeds**) may occur.

💡 **What to Do:**

✔ Apply **firm pressure** to stop bleeding.

✔ Use a **soft toothbrush** and **electric razor** to avoid irritation.

✔ Avoid **high-impact activities** that could cause injuries.

🚨 **Call a doctor if bleeding does not stop within 10–15 minutes.**

Serious Side Effects (When to Call a Doctor)

While rare, some side effects of Enoxaparin can be serious and require **immediate medical attention**.

1. Signs of Internal Bleeding

🚨 Seek medical help immediately if you experience:

❗ **Unusual bruising** (large, unexplained, or worsening bruises).

❗ **Dark, tarry stools** or blood in urine.

❗ **Coughing up blood** or severe nosebleeds.

❗ **Severe headaches, dizziness, or confusion** (possible brain bleed).

💡 **Internal bleeding can be dangerous—never ignore these symptoms.**

2. Allergic Reactions (Rare but Serious)

Some people may have an **allergic reaction** to Enoxaparin.

🚨 Call emergency services if you experience:

❗ **Swelling of the face, lips, or throat**.

❗ **Difficulty breathing** or wheezing.

❗ **Severe rash, itching, or hives**.

💡 **If you have a known allergy to heparin-based drugs, inform your doctor before starting Enoxaparin.**

Managing Side Effects at Home

Most mild side effects can be managed with **simple home remedies**:

✔ **For bruising or pain:** Apply a **cold compress** after injection.
✔ **For mild bleeding:** Use **gentle pressure** and avoid blood-thinning foods (like garlic, ginger, and fish oil).
✔ **For mild dizziness:** Stand up **slowly** from sitting or lying positions.
✔ **For minor skin irritation:** Keep **injection sites clean and dry**, and switch to a **different site** each time.

🚨 **Always consult your doctor before stopping or adjusting your Enoxaparin dose.**

Key Takeaways

✔ **Mild side effects (bruising, minor bleeding) are common and manageable.**
✔ **Serious symptoms (internal bleeding, allergic reactions) require immediate medical attention.**
✔ **Proper injection techniques can minimize pain and irritation.**
✔ **Monitor for unusual bleeding and contact a doctor if symptoms worsen.**

Chapter 5:

Warnings and Precautions

While Enoxaparin (Clexane) is a highly effective medication for preventing and treating blood clots, it may not be suitable for everyone. Certain medical conditions, medications, and lifestyle factors can increase the risk of complications. This chapter outlines who should avoid Enoxaparin, important drug interactions, and necessary lifestyle adjustments to ensure safe use.

Who Should Avoid Enoxaparin?

Certain individuals should **not take Enoxaparin** or must use it with extreme caution. Always consult your doctor before starting treatment if you have any of the following conditions:

1. Allergies to Enoxaparin or Heparin-Based Medications

Do **not** use Enoxaparin if you have had a severe **allergic reaction** to:

❌ **Enoxaparin (Clexane), Heparin, or other low molecular weight heparins (LMWHs).**

❌ **Benzyl alcohol (a preservative found in multi-dose vials of Enoxaparin).**

Symptoms of an allergic reaction include:

- Swelling of the face, lips, or throat
- Severe itching or hives
- Difficulty breathing

2. Bleeding Disorders or High Bleeding Risk

Since Enoxaparin is a **blood thinner**, it can increase the risk of **excessive bleeding**. You should **avoid or use it with caution** if you have:

❗ **Hemophilia or other clotting disorders**
❗ **Active stomach ulcers or gastrointestinal bleeding**
❗ **A history of brain bleeds or hemorrhagic strokes**

Your doctor may need to adjust your dose or recommend an alternative medication.

---

3. Recent Surgeries or Medical Procedures

Enoxaparin may increase the risk of **post-surgical bleeding,** especially in:

🩺 **Recent brain, spine, or eye surgery**
🩺 **Uncontrolled high blood pressure**
🩺 **Patients with an epidural or spinal catheter** (risk of spinal bleeding and paralysis)

If you need surgery while on Enoxaparin, inform your doctor beforehand to adjust your treatment plan.

Drug Interactions

Certain medications can **increase the risk of bleeding** or reduce the effectiveness of Enoxaparin.

Medications to Avoid (or Use with Caution)

🚨 **High-risk drug interactions include:**
❌ **Aspirin (unless prescribed by your doctor)**
❌ **NSAIDs (e.g., Ibuprofen, Naproxen, Diclofenac) – can increase bleeding risk**
❌ **Other anticoagulants (e.g., Warfarin, Rivaroxaban, Apixaban)**
❌ **Clopidogrel (Plavix) and other antiplatelet drugs**
❌ **Herbal supplements (e.g., Ginkgo biloba, Garlic, Fish oil) – can thin blood further**

💡 **Always inform your doctor about all medications, including over-the-counter drugs and supplements.**

Lifestyle Adjustments

Taking Enoxaparin requires some **lifestyle changes** to minimize the risk of injury or excessive bleeding.

1. Alcohol Use

❗ **Alcohol can increase the risk of bleeding** because it affects blood clotting.

💡 **Tips for Safe Alcohol Use:**
✔ Avoid **heavy drinking** (can worsen bruising and bleeding).
✔ If drinking, **limit to 1-2 drinks occasionally** and monitor for unusual bruising or bleeding.

---

2. Sports and Physical Activities

Since Enoxaparin increases bleeding risk, certain activities should be **avoided or modified**.

❌ **High-risk sports (avoid due to injury risk):**

- **Contact sports** (football, rugby, boxing)
- **Extreme sports** (skiing, skydiving)
- **Heavy weightlifting** (can cause internal bleeding)

✅ **Safer activities (low-impact exercises):**

- Walking or light jogging
- Yoga and stretching
- Swimming and cycling

If you experience unusual bruising or pain after exercise, stop and consult your doctor.

---

3. Injury Prevention

Because Enoxaparin makes it **harder for blood to clot**, even minor injuries can lead to excessive bleeding.

◆ **Safety Tips:**

✔ Use **a soft-bristled toothbrush** to prevent gum bleeding.
✔ Shave with **an electric razor** instead of blades.
✔ Be **cautious with sharp objects** (e.g., knives, scissors).
✔ Wear **protective gear** if working in a high-risk environment.

🚨 Seek immediate medical attention if you experience severe bleeding, large unexplained bruises, or head injuries.

Key Takeaways

✔ Avoid Enoxaparin if you have severe allergies, bleeding disorders, or recent brain/spine surgery.

✔ Avoid medications that increase bleeding risk, such as NSAIDs and aspirin.

✔ Limit alcohol consumption and avoid contact sports or high-impact activities.

✔ Take extra precautions to prevent injuries and minimize bleeding risks.

Chapter 6:

Special Populations

Enoxaparin (Clexane) is commonly prescribed for **pregnant women, elderly patients, and, in rare cases, children**. However, its use in these groups requires **careful monitoring and dosage adjustments**. This chapter covers how Enoxaparin is used in these special populations, including **precautions, safety concerns, and key recommendations**.

Is Enoxaparin Safe During Pregnancy?

✅ **Yes, Enoxaparin is widely used during pregnancy** for conditions that increase the risk of blood clots, such as:

- **Preventing pregnancy loss in women with thrombophilia** (e.g., antiphospholipid syndrome, Factor V Leiden).
- **Treating deep vein thrombosis (DVT) or pulmonary embolism (PE) during pregnancy.**
- **Preventing blood clots in high-risk pregnancies, such as those involving IVF or a history of clotting disorders.**

💡 **Unlike Warfarin, Enoxaparin does not cross the placenta**, making it safer for the baby.

How Is Enoxaparin Used in Pregnancy?

🩺 **Dose Adjustments:** A doctor may adjust the dosage **as pregnancy progresses**, especially in the third trimester.

🗓 **Stopping Before Delivery:** Enoxaparin is often **stopped 24–36 hours before labor** to reduce the risk of excessive bleeding. 💉 **Switching to Heparin:** Some women may be switched to **unfractionated heparin** closer to delivery for easier reversal if needed.

Is Enoxaparin Safe During Breastfeeding?

✅ **Yes, Enoxaparin is considered safe for breastfeeding mothers** because:

- **Minimal amounts** pass into breast milk.
- No harmful effects have been reported in breastfed infants.

💡 **Mothers taking Enoxaparin can continue breastfeeding safely.**

Use in Elderly Patients

As people age, their bodies **process medications differently**, and elderly patients may be at a **higher risk of bleeding**. Enoxaparin is commonly prescribed to older adults for conditions like **DVT, PE, and post-surgical clot prevention** but requires special considerations.

Key Precautions for Elderly Patients:

✔ **Kidney Function Monitoring:** Enoxaparin is cleared through the **kidneys**, so doctors may **reduce the dose** in patients with kidney disease.

✔ **Bleeding Risk Assessment:** Older adults may be more prone to **bruising, internal bleeding, or falls**, so close monitoring is essential.

✔ **Fall Prevention:** Since excessive bleeding can be dangerous, elderly patients should **take extra precautions to avoid falls or injuries**.

Elderly patients should have regular check-ups to monitor kidney function and bleeding risks while on Enoxaparin.

Paediatric Use (Rare Cases)

Is Enoxaparin Used in Children?

Yes, but only in rare cases and under close medical supervision. Enoxaparin may be prescribed for children with:

- **Congenital clotting disorders.**
- **Post-surgical clot prevention (e.g., after heart surgery).**
- **Blood clot conditions linked to prolonged immobility or certain diseases.**

How Is Enoxaparin Used in Children?

Dosing is weight-based and carefully calculated by a pediatric specialist.

Frequent blood tests are required to monitor the drug's effects.

Infants and small children may receive injections in the thigh instead of the abdomen for easier administration.

Because data on Enoxaparin use in children is limited, it is only used when absolutely necessary.

Key Takeaways

✔ **Enoxaparin is safe and widely used during pregnancy and breastfeeding.**

✔ **In elderly patients, dosage adjustments may be needed to prevent excessive bleeding.**

✔ **Enoxaparin is rarely used in children and requires close monitoring by a specialist.**

Chapter 7:

Managing Enoxaparin Day-to-Day

Taking Enoxaparin (Clexane) as part of your daily routine requires **careful management** to ensure safety and effectiveness. This chapter provides answers to common questions, tips for living with Enoxaparin, a quick reference chart for doses and side effects, an injection site rotation diagram, and a sample medication diary to help you stay organized.

Frequently Asked Questions

1. How long do I need to take Enoxaparin?

The duration of Enoxaparin treatment depends on your condition:

- **DVT/PE Treatment:** Usually **3–6 months**.
- **Pregnancy-Related Use:** Often **until 6 weeks postpartum**.
- **Post-Surgery Prevention:** Typically **7–10 days**, but sometimes longer.

Your doctor will determine the exact duration based on your health needs.

2. What should I do if I miss a dose?

- **If it's been a few hours**, take the missed dose as soon as possible.
- **If it's close to the next dose,** skip the missed dose—**do not double-dose.**

- **Set reminders** to help prevent missed doses.

3. Can I stop taking Enoxaparin suddenly?

No! Stopping suddenly can **increase the risk of blood clots**. Always consult your doctor before discontinuing.

4. What happens if I inject into the wrong site?

If you accidentally inject into a **bruised, painful, or unsuitable area**, don't panic:

✔ Choose a different injection site next time.

✔ Monitor for **unusual swelling, pain, or bleeding**.

✔ If in doubt, consult your doctor.

5. Can I travel while taking Enoxaparin?

Yes! But take precautions:

✔ Carry a **doctor's prescription and medical note** if traveling by air.

✔ Keep Enoxaparin in its **original packaging** to avoid issues at security.

✔ Store syringes at the correct temperature (not in direct sunlight or extreme cold).

Living with Enoxaparin

Taking Enoxaparin long-term requires **a few lifestyle adjustments**:

◆ **Daily Routine Tips:**

✔ Set a **fixed time** for injections to maintain consistency.

✔ Rotate injection sites to avoid irritation and bruising.

✔ Keep a **medication diary** (see sample below) to track doses.

◆ **Exercise and Activity:**

✔ Stick to **low-impact** activities like walking and swimming.

✖ Avoid **contact sports** or activities with a high risk of injury.

◆ **Bleeding Precautions:**

✔ Use a **soft-bristled toothbrush** to prevent gum bleeding.

✔ Shave with an **electric razor** instead of a blade.

✔ Be **careful with sharp objects** like knives and scissors.

Quick Reference Chart (Doses, Side Effects, Emergency Contacts)

Condition	Typical Dose	Duration
DVT/PE Treatment	1 mg/kg **twice daily** or 1.5 mg/kg **once daily**	3–6 months
Pregnancy	40 mg **once daily** (may vary)	Until **6 weeks postpartum**
Post-Surgery	40 mg **once daily**	7–10 days
Heart Conditions (e.g., angina)	1 mg/kg **twice daily**	As prescribed

Emergency Contact Signs (Call a doctor immediately if you experience):

- **Excessive bruising or prolonged bleeding**
- **Dark stools or blood in urine**
- **Severe headache or dizziness** (possible internal bleeding)

📞 **Emergency Contacts:**

- **Doctor's Name: __________________**
- **Hospital/Clinic: __________________**
- **Emergency Helpline: ______________**

Injection Site Rotation Diagram

To **reduce pain, bruising, and irritation**, it's important to rotate injection sites.

Recommended Injection Areas:

✔ **Abdomen (preferred site)** – At least **2 inches away from the belly button**

✔ **Thighs (front or outer thigh)**

✔ **Upper arms (less common, but possible)**

Rotation Schedule Example:

- **Day 1:** Left abdomen
- **Day 2:** Right abdomen
- **Day 3:** Left thigh

- **Day 4:** Right thigh
- **Day 5:** Repeat cycle

💡 **Tip:** Avoid injecting into **bruised or irritated areas**!

Sample Medication Diary

📖 **Keeping a medication diary** helps you track doses and identify any unusual side effects.

Date	Time	Injection Site	Any Side Effects?
01/03/2025	8:00 AM	Left Abdomen	Mild bruising
02/03/2025	8:00 AM	Right Abdomen	No issues
03/03/2025	8:00 AM	Left Thigh	Small swelling
04/03/2025	8:00 AM	Right Thigh	No issues

💡 **Tip:** Take this log to your doctor's visits for better monitoring!

Key Takeaways

✔ **Stay consistent** with your injection routine.
✔ **Use the rotation schedule** to prevent bruising.
✔ **Keep a quick reference chart** handy for dosing and emergency contacts.
✔ **Log daily injections** to track your response to the medication.

NOTES

ABOUT THE AUTHOR

Asharani Sah is a dedicated medical writer and researcher with a deep passion for advancing knowledge in **obstetrics, gynaecology, and reproductive medicine**. With years of experience in **medical literature review, clinical research, and evidence-based writing**, her specializes in translating complex medical concepts into clear, practical guidance for healthcare professionals.

Her work focuses on providing **scientifically rigorous, well-researched, and clinically relevant** insights into topics such as **pregnancy care, hormonal therapies, and fertility treatments**. Committed to bridging the gap between research and practice, she ensures that medical professionals have access to the most **up-to-date and reliable information** to support patient care.

When not immersed in medical literature, Asharani enjoys exploring emerging trends in pharmacology, attending medical conferences, and contributing to professional discussions on **women's health and reproductive endocrinology**.

This book, **"Enoxaparin (Clexane) and Pregnancy: How Necessary and Safe Is It?"**, is a testament to his commitment to **delivering high-quality, evidence-based medical knowledge** to practitioners worldwide.

We Value Your Feedback!

If you found this book helpful, please consider leaving a rating and sharing your thoughts. Your feedback not only guides other readers to find practical, reliable information but also helps Mrs Asharani to continually improve her work based on your needs.

Whether it's a brief comment or a detailed review, your feedback will make a difference. Thank you for helping us make this guide a valuable resource for everyone!

www.ingramcontent.com/pod-product-compliance
Ingram Content Group UK Ltd.
Pitfield, Milton Keynes, MK11 3LW, UK
UKHW021342190726
13845UKWH00027B/681

9 789334 246797